SMOOTHIES THAT HEAL!

Your Key to Optimal Health!

Valerie Ramdin

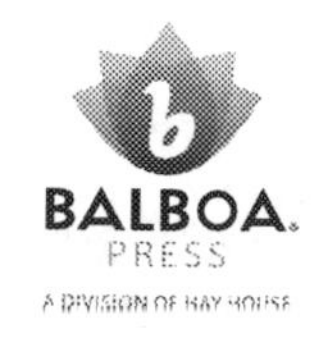

Author Credits: PhD. Counselling

Balboa Press books may be ordered through booksellers or by contacting:

Balboa Press
A Division of Hay House
1663 Liberty Drive
Bloomington, IN 47403
www.balboapress.com
1-(877) 407-4847

Printed in the United States of America.

ISBN: 978-1-4525-7218-5 (sc)
ISBN: 978-1-4525-7219-2 (e)

Balboa Press rev. date: 04/22/2013

I would like to thank my family and friends for their constant support: Joshua Wesson, Patricia Ramdin, Jacalyn Johnson, Clete Ramdin, Ruby Ray, and Bernard Aleman.

Smoothies that heal!
Easy!
Delicious!
Healthy!
Fortified with Superfoods!

Table of Contents

What do I Know?

In October of 1993, I was diagnosed with Multiple Sclerosis. In October of 2010, I started my own healing program and in December 2011, I was taken off all MS medication with doctor's approval. It took me one year to get off all medications and have no symptoms! I am sharing the smoothie recipes that I use to maintain my symptom-free life. With MS, I experienced the following symptoms: extreme muscle weakness, slurring of speech, optic neuritis, detached retina, migraines, weak core muscles, muscle spasms, limb paralysis, fatigue, dizziness and more. I am sharing these recipes with the hope that you will use them to recover and revitalize your health. Today, I run 4 miles or more a day and enjoy a full life with no medical constraints. Please share these recipes with your loved ones as a preventive measure. Oh yes, what's even more; I learned that the tips I discovered; not only improve my chronic health condition, but also improve many other chronic health conditions!!

Why Smoothies?

I drink two smoothies a day. Why not just eat the fruit? Well, when vegetables are blended into a pulp, incredible nutrients are released that you can only get by masticating(chewing) over and over again. Most vitamins pills are made of fruit and vegetables. Most of us miss these nutrients by eating too quickly. Or not chewing enough. Or not eating enough of the right thing. Vitamins alone are not as effective as a proper diet. By cooking veggies and fruit, the vitamins and nutrients are reduced by variable amounts, according to the documentary, "Food Matters" with David Wolfe. Therefore, it makes perfect sense to reinforce your daily vitamin intake with healthy raw fruit and vegetables.

Where Should You Start

I like to use a blender instead of a juicer; because, I have gained tremendous results from eating the entire fruit and vegetable. Besides the fiber is important! By combining fruit and veggies; you can have healthy and delicious drinks.

I purchase fresh fruit on sale and wash it with homemade veggie wash (sea salt or vinegar solution). I use a select list of anti-inflammatory veggies and fruit. I also make sure that the produce is anti-angiogenic as well. Dr. William Li has such lists posted on the internet under (http://www.ted.com/talks/william_li.html).

Improvement is the Key

By improving my eating habits, exercising regularly, meditating daily, and fostering a positive attitude; I no longer experience any of the symptoms of multiple sclerosis that I was diagnosed with approximately 20 years ago! I was taken off of the MS medical treatment completely. I had gained weight using the MS medication and could not even exercise without throwing myself into a relapse! And my gosh! The symptoms I experienced from the medication really dropped my quality of life also. Taking the medication, I could not exercise daily or I would relapse back into those symptoms! I would get really stressed at work and I would go into a relapse! I would get stressed with my personal life and I would relapse! My bladder was shot at 35 years old!? What?? I determined that the medication was effective for "emergency "management of my symptoms; however, the long term use was making me miserable!

Your Turn

I would like to share some of my favorite recipes with you. I drink these smoothies twice daily as an integral part of my personal health plan! If I am hungry or wanting a snack ; I make a smoothie. I made these smoothies extra tasty. I enjoy the smoothies without the apple juice whatsoever! I exclude the apple juice to avoid unnecessary weight gain and complications from the concentrated fructose or fruit sugar. But if you and your loved ones have no problems with natural fruit juice; then enjoy them with the apple juice**. I prepare the smoothies for myself and son with skim milk or water. My first benefit was improved digestion!** I get noticeable benefits from the *Super Effective* healing variation in the "Punch It Up" section!

So Simple

Remember garbage in . . . . garbage out! If you put garbage in your body it will come out in different "garbagy" ways like sickness . . . . disease and other various conditions! Put in simple whole foods to strengthen your body and restore.

Oh my gosh . . . Could it be that simple? Yes. It is that simple. Choose to be strong and healthy! Skip the fast food and processed foods. Fast food is made to make financial profit. When a meal is prepared from scratch using no processed ingredients, it can be prepared to be tasty and nurturing.

I know that there are some fast food exceptions like your local fast smoothie shops; but in general, fast food should be avoided.

I have created some recipes with some fruit that are easily accessible. This book is comprised of different recipes that combined fruit and vegetables to create a variety of different tastes. All of the recipes are anti-cancerous, anti-inflammatory, heart strengthening recipes. What is so incredible is that these "life-giving" foods are always within our reach!! These nutrient rich smoothies also promote improved energy and skin! Let your doctor know that you are making smoothies from fruit and vegetables every day. Now, prepare to be amazed!

Twenty Recipes

CHOOSE GREAT HEALTH!! It has never been easier!!!

Simply Grapes

1 cup of red seedless grapes
6 oz natural apple juice (no sweetener added)
6 oz ice water or ice

ADD INGREDIENTS TO BLENDER AND BLEND AT HIGH SPEED FOR ONE MINUTE.

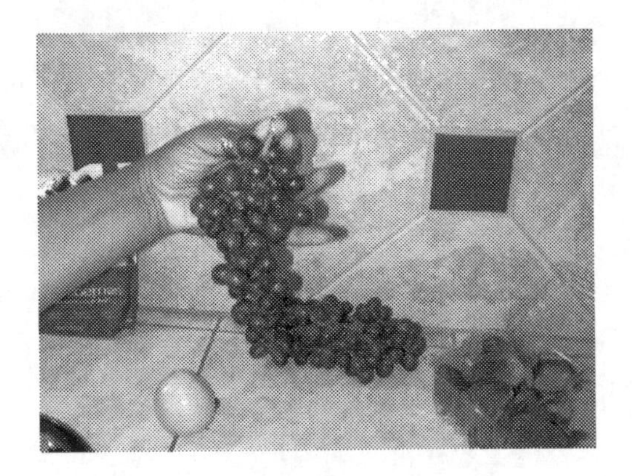

Notes: ______________________________

PUNCH IT UP:

Add ¼ tsp of vanilla flavoring for more flavor!
Add ¼ tsp of cinnamon for anti-inflammatory aid.
Add 1tsp-1TBSN of olive oil to create a digestive aid!
Add I TBSPN of honey for ENERGY!
Substitute soy milk or skim or nut milk for a variation!

SUPER EFFECTIVE HEALING: Use water instead of apple juice and add one serving of spirulina powder and wheatgrass powder (or wheatgrass shot).

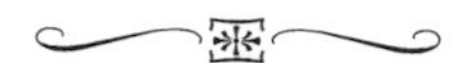

WHAT EXCITES ME ABOUT THIS ONE!: Grapes are known for being anti-inflammatory/anti-cancerous due to health strengthening agent: resveratrol. There are many more benefits of the grape found at organicfacts.net. This drink also regulates the bowels. It improves skin diseases and acne. The apple juice also aids in digestion. It has potassium which strengthens the heart, muscular skeletal system, respiratory system, nervous system and more.

This simple drink is chocked full of magnesium, potassium, zinc and other vital minerals that can stop diseases and improve over-all health. Most of my smoothies have vegetables-but; this one is so simple and powerful, that people have claimed to stop cancer with it. I know personally, this drink has stopped my adult acne breakouts. But, I eat very little processed sugar for best results. If you cannot cut out the processed sugar products, then limit them.

Grape Ape

1 Banana
½ cup of dark or red grapes
4 oz apple juice
4 oz ice water
¼ teaspoon of cinnamon

ADD INGREDIENTS TO BLENDER AND BLEND AT HIGH SPEED FOR ONE MINUTE.
BENEFITS: This is a totally anti-inflammatory, anti cancer, drink.

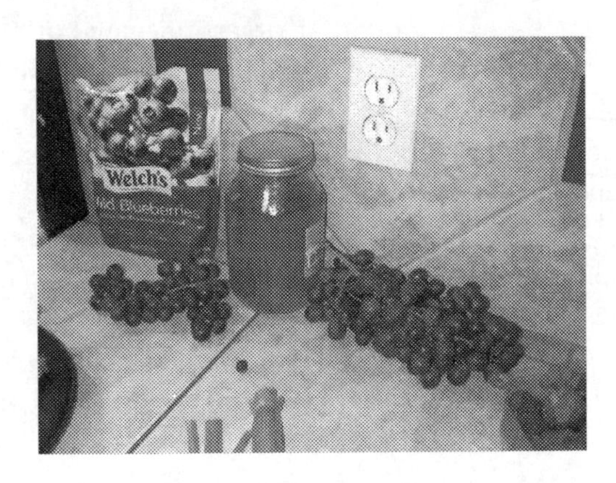

Notes: ______________________________

____

____

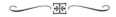

PUNCH IT UP:

Add ¼ tsp of vanilla flavoring for more flavor!
Add 1tsp-1TBSN of olive oil to create a digestive aid!
Add 1 TBSPN of honey of ENERGY!
Substitute soy milk or skim or nut milk for apple juice for a creamy variation!

SUPER EFFECTIVE HEALING: Use water instead of apple juice and add one serving of spirulina powder and wheatgrass powder (or wheatgrass shot).

WHAT EXCITES ME ABOUT THIS ONE: Wow, I love this one! The grapes are so medicinal. They will keep you *regular* and with the combination of the banana and the apple juice. Grapes are used also to get rid of migraines! Have fun with this recipe. APPLE JUICE IS GREAT!!!! Apples have so many benefits. These fruit are anti-inflammatory, fibre-rich, vitamin and mineral rich gold mines in the fruit arena! The cinnamon reduces inflammation also and strengthens the heart! There are no green "leafies" in this one; I exchanged them for an apple that is fibre-rich and chocked full of anti-oxidants also, so remember your kale smoothie or salad later on today!!!! YOU GO!! HAVE A BEAUTIFUL DAY!!!!!!

Kale/Grape blast

1 cup of kale (or raw collard greens)
½ cup red seedless grapes
8 ice oz water
5 oz apple juice

ADD INGREDIENTS TO BLENDER AND BLEND AT HIGH SPEED FOR ONE MINUTE.

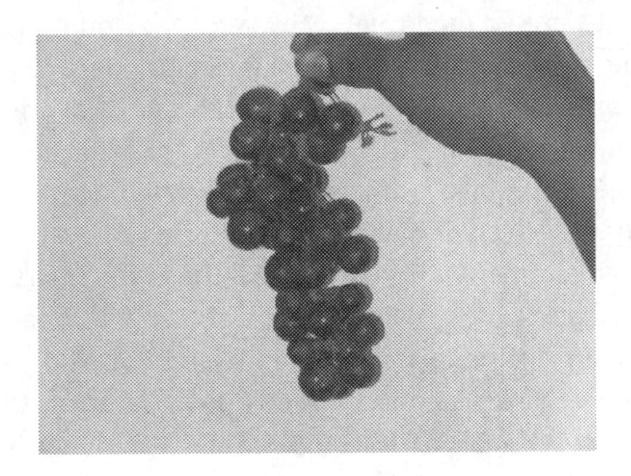

Notes: ____

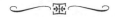

PUNCH IT UP:

Add ¼ tsp of vanilla flavoring for more flavor!
Add ¼ tsp of cinnamon for anti-inflammatory aid.
Add 1tsp-1TBSN of olive oil to create a digestive aid!
Substitute soy milk, low-fat milk, almond milk for a creamy variation.

SUPER EFFECTIVE HEALING: Use water instead of apple juice and add one serving of spirulina powder and wheatgrass powder (or wheatgrass shot).

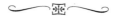

WHAT EXCITES ME ABOUT THIS ONE: Kale! KALE!! KALE. KALE is anti-inflammatory and great for the digestion. There is a reason that KALE is a superfood! It has important vitamins and minerals that build a healthy muscular-skeletal foundation . . . . not to mention it helps with your beautiful skin!! Add that to the grapes and apple juice and you have a real beauty potion and digestive aid and overall super-health tonic!! Don't you feel great just reading bout that one. GREAT DRINK! GREAT DAY!!!

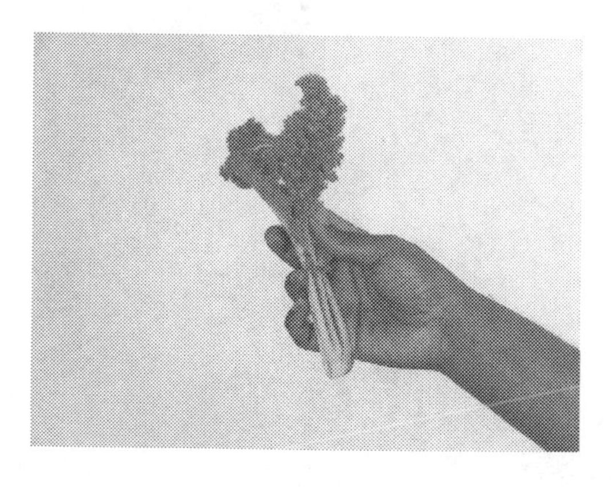

Radiant Skin Drink

1 cup of kale (or raw collard greens)
½ cup of grapes (dark or red)
½ banana
5 oz ice water
5 oz apple juice
¼ tsp cinnamon

ADD INGREDIENTS TO BLENDER AND BLEND AT HIGH SPEED FOR ONE MINUTE.

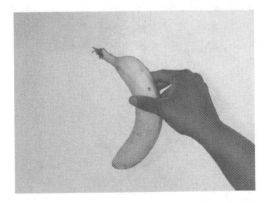

Notes: ____

____

____

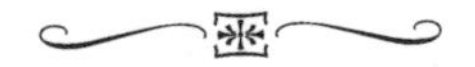

PUNCH IT UP:

Add ¼ tsp vanilla to this one for intense flavor!
EXCHANGE 1 cup crushed ice for apple juice to make a treat!
Add ¼ tsp of vanilla flavoring for more flavor
Add 1tsp-1TBSN of olive oil to create a digestive aid!

SUPER EFFECTIVE HEALING: Use water instead of apple juice and add one serving of spirulina powder and wheatgrass powder (or wheatgrass shot).

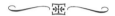

WHAT EXCITES ME ABOUT THIS RECIPE: Kale is a superfood—full of vital minerals and vitamins along with dark grapes that are an anti-cancer, anti-inflammatory produce as well. The banana and apple juice help with digestion and flavor!! YUM. The cinnamon and nutmeg help with strengthening the heart. Cinnamon is anti-inflammatory. ANOTHER HIT! YOU ARE DOING IT RIGHT WITH THIS ONE!!!

Apple/Grapes blend

6 or 7 grapes
1 small quartered apple
5 oz ice water
5 oz apple juice
¼ tsp vanilla flavoring

ADD INGREDIENTS TO BLENDER AND BLEND AT HIGH SPEED FOR ONE MINUTE.

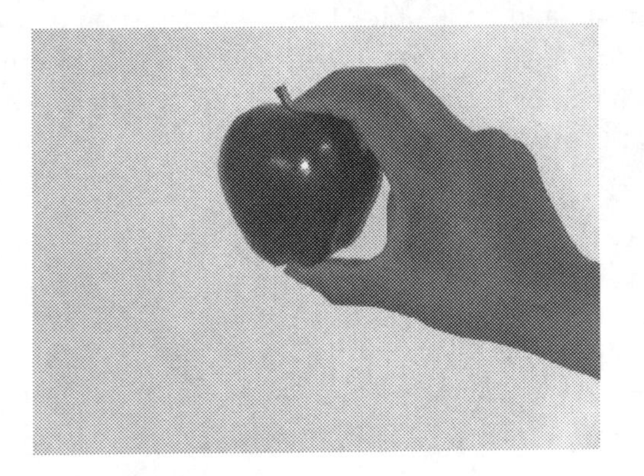

Notes: ____

____

____

____

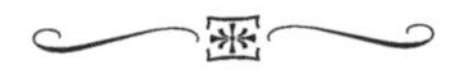

PUNCH IT UP:

Add 1tsp-1TBSN of olive oil to create a digestive aid!
Add 1 TBSPN of honey of ENERGY!
Substitute soy milk or skim or nut milk for apple juice and water for variation!
Add ¼ tsp of cinnamon for anti-inflammatory aid.
Add 1tsp-1TBSN of olive oil to create a digestive aid!

SUPER EFFECTIVE HEALING: Use water instead of apple juice and add one serving of spirulina powder and wheatgrass powder (or wheatgrass shot).

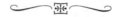

WHAT EXCITES ME ABOUT THIS RECIPE: Grapes are yummy and full of anti-cancerous anti-inflammatory agents. The apples help so much with digestion and they are also anti-inflammatory. This smoothie contains vital nutrients and isanti-cancerous. It is filling and tasty. The vanilla makes this smoothie pop!!! *Another GREAT SKIN SMOOTHIE!!*

Apple/Cinnamon Breakfast

1 sm quartered apple
¼ tsp cinnamon
1 heaping tablespoon peanut butter (or any other nut butter)
1 tablespoon honey
5 oz apple juice
5 oz ice water

ADD INGREDIENTS TO BLENDER AND BLEND AT HIGH SPEED FOR ONE MINUTE

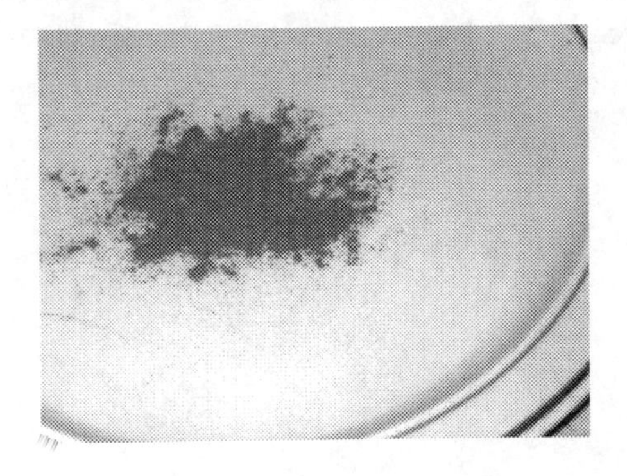

Notes: ______________________________

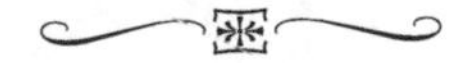

PUNCH IT UP:

Add ¼ tsp of vanilla flavoring for more flavor!
Add ¼ tsp of cinnamon for anti-inflammatory aid.
Add 1tsp-1TBSN of olive oil to create a digestive aid!

SUPER EFFECTIVE HEALING: Use water instead of apple juice and add one serving of spirulina powder and wheatgrass powder (or wheatgrass shot).

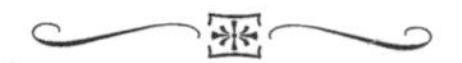

WHAT EXCITES ME ABOUT THIS RECIPE: This one is filling and will take you farther than cereal or a donut! The honey and cinnamon along with the nut butter make you want to run to work. Cinnamon is heart strengthening and anti-inflammatory coupled with the all-time champion APPLE that holds the title for being antioxidant/fibre fruit! The peanut butter adds the protein and oil component that takes this drink over the edge for maintaining strong muscles and bones! This is a tasty light breakfast or snack that satisfies the stomach for hours!

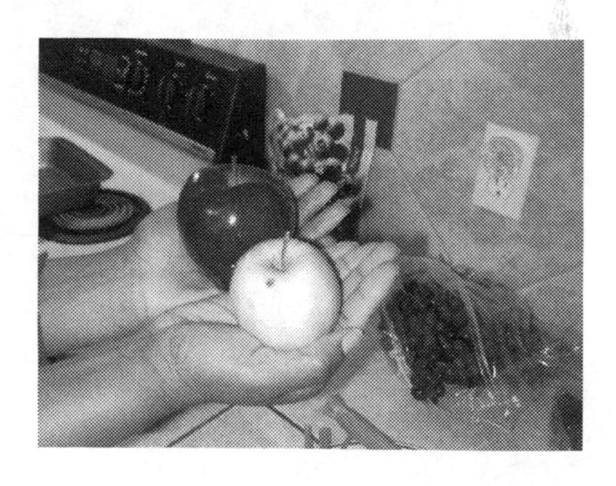

Kale/Peanut butter blend

1 cup kale (or raw collard greens)
1 tablespoon peanut butter (or nut butter: cashew, almond etc.)
1 cup ice cold apple juice
½ cup ice water

ADD INGREDIENTS TO BLENDER AND BLEND AT HIGH SPEED FOR ONE MINUTE.

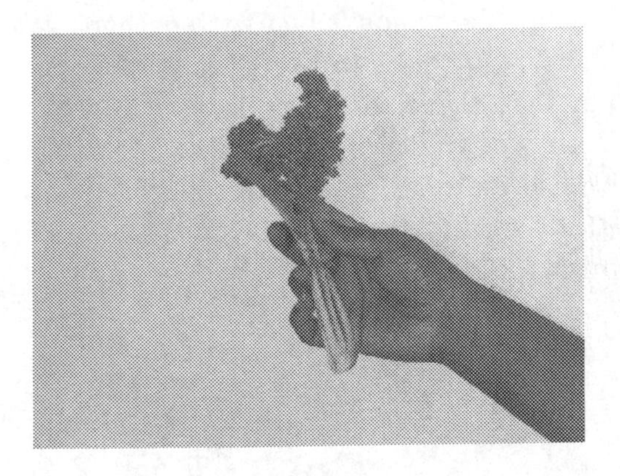

Notes

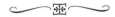

PUNCH IT UP:

Add ¼ tsp of vanilla flavoring for more flavor!
Add 1tsp-1TBSN of olive oil to create a digestive aid!
Add I TBSPN of honey of ENERGY!
Substitute soy milk or skim or nut milk for a variation!

SUPER EFFECTIVE HEALING: Use water instead of apple j and add one serving of spirulina powder and wheatgr powder (or wheatgrass shot).

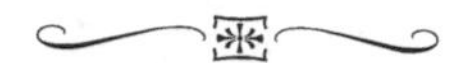

WHAT EXCITES ME ABOUT THIS RECIPE: The nut butter helps especially before your morning run or work-out. The kale is a wonderful super food that helps with digestion. The apple makes it taste good and whole drink is chock full of anti-inflammatory /anti-cancer ingredients! The kale has vitamins and minerals that will help cleanse your system resulting in improved overall health. By consuming anti-inflammatory KALE (or other such greens) daily in the raw form, you improve your overall health!

Apple to Oranges

1 small orange (clementines or tangerines work great!)
1 quartered sm apple
1 dash cinnamon
½ cup apple juice
½ cup ice water

ADD INGREDIENTS TO BLENDER AND BLEND AT HIGH SPEED FOR ONE MINUTE.

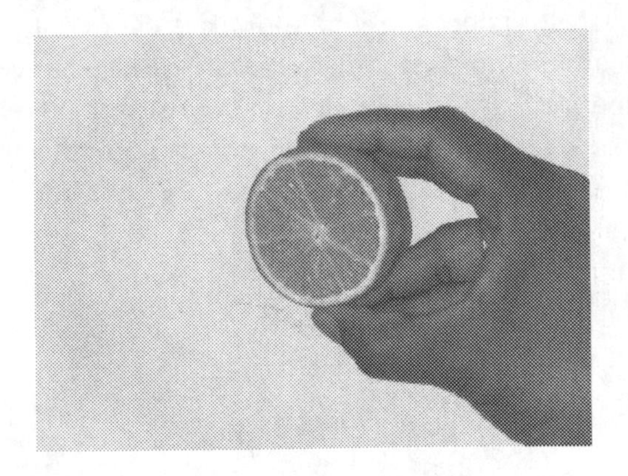

Notes: ______________________________

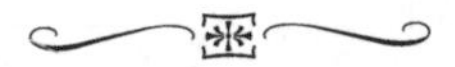

PUNCH IT UP:

Add ¼ tsp of vanilla flavoring for more flavor!
Add ¼ tsp of cinnamon for anti-inflammatory aid.
Add 1tsp-1TBSN of olive oil to create a digestive aid!

SUPER EFFECTIVE HEALING: Use water instead of apple juice and add one serving of spirulina powder and wheatgrass powder (or wheatgrass shot).

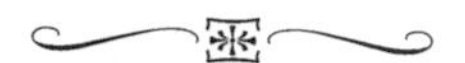

WHAT EXCITES ME ABOUT THIS RECIPE: The oranges are anti-cancerous and anti-inflammatory; the apples are great for digestion and are anti-oxidants as well as full of health building agents that lower cholesterol and strengthen the immune system etc. They are tasty!! This drink is healthy and tasty. What doesn't excite you about this one?
Have a tremendous day!!! Yeah . . . . Tremendous!

Orange squared

1 small orange (clementine or tangerines work best)
1 chopped carrot
1 dash cinnamon
½ cup apple juice
½ water

ADD INGREDIENTS TO BLENDER AND BLEND AT HIGH SPEED FOR ONE MINUTE.

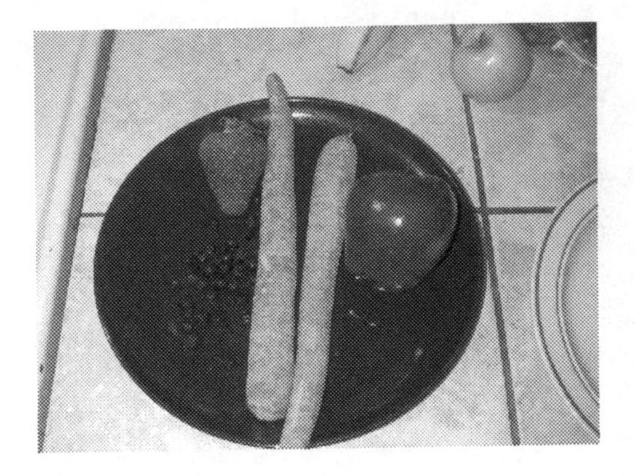

Notes:____

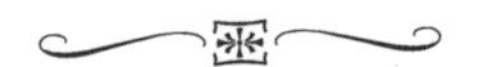

PUNCH IT UP:

Add ¼ tsp of vanilla flavoring for more flavor!
Add 1tsp-1TBSN of olive oil to create a digestive aid!
Add 1 TBSPN of honey of ENERGY!
Substitute soy milk or skim or nut milk for a variation!

SUPER EFFECTIVE HEALING: Use water instead of apple juice and add one serving of spirulina powder and wheatgrass powder (or wheatgrass shot).

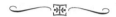

WHAT EXCITES ME ABOUT THIS RECIPE: This is a great drink. The carrots provide a filling drink that tastes great. The fiber helps with digestion and of course this one is great for your skin!!! It is anti-cancerous and anti-inflammatory. Carrots are so great for your digestion! **Check with your doctor. I read that blending fruit with carrots can promote goiters in some. I have eaten carrots blended with fruit quite often with no such effects; I checked with my doctor.**

Toss UP

1 banana
1 small orange
1 apple
1 cup kale (or raw collard greens)
6 oz apple juice
6 oz ice water
¼ tsp cinnamon

ADD INGREDIENTS TO BLENDER AND BLEND AT HIGH SPEED FOR ONE MINUTE.

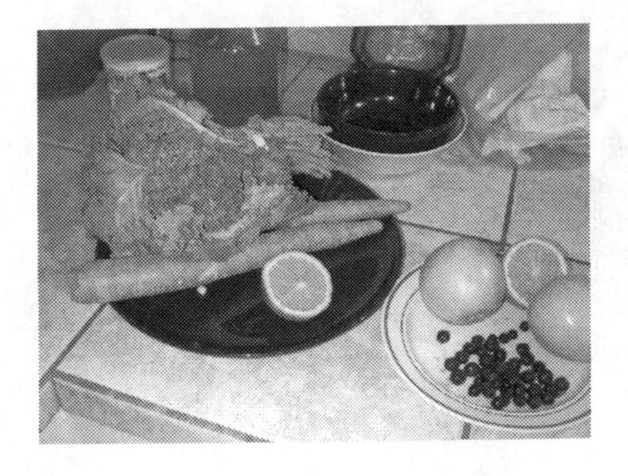

Notes: ______________________________

____

____

____

____

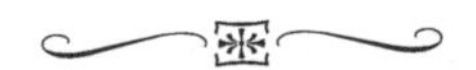

PUNCH IT UP:

Add 1tsp-1TBSN of olive oil to create a digestive aid!
Add 1 TBSPN of honey of ENERGY!
Substitute soy milk or skim or nut milk for a variation!

SUPER EFFECTIVE HEALING: Use water instead of apple juice and add one serving of spirulina powder and wheatgrass powder (or wheatgrass shot).

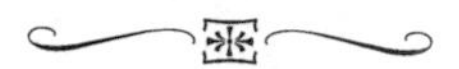

WHAT EXCITES ME ABOUT THIS RECIPE: This one is filling and chock full of anti-cancerous/ anti-inflammatory fruit and veggies. WOW!! The apple, orange and kale are all anti-inflammatory. Cinnamon is also anti-inflammatory. All the fruit in this drink is anti-cancerous as well.

Apple-Kale-Banana Blend

1 quartered apple
1 cup kale (or raw collard greens)
1 banana
1 cup of apple juice
1 cup of ice water
¼ tsp vanilla

ADD INGREDIENTS TO BLENDER AND BLEND AT HIGH SPEED FOR ONE MINUTE.

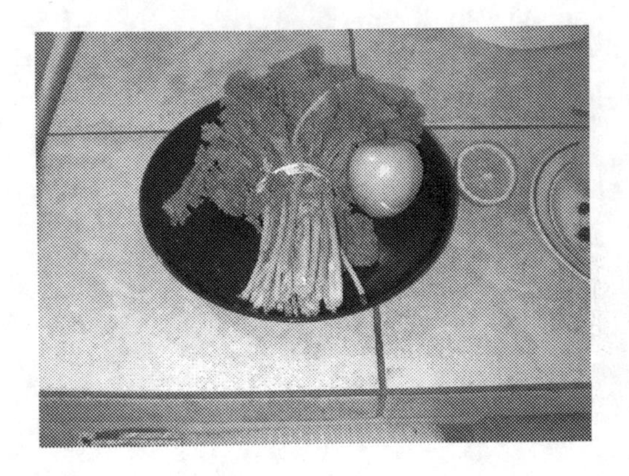

Notes:

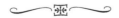

PUNCH IT UP:

Add ¼ tsp of cinnamon for flavor and anti-inflammatory aid!
Add 1tsp-1TBSN of olive oil to create a digestive aid!
Add 1 TBSPN of honey of ENERGY!
Substitute soy milk or skim or nut milk for a variation!

SUPER EFFECTIVE HEALING: Use water instead of apple juice and add one serving of spirulina powder and wheatgrass powder (or wheatgrass shot).

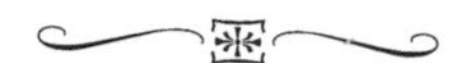

WHAT EXCITES ME ABOUT THIS RECIPE: This is a delicious recipe full of anti-cancerous fruit. The vanilla and banana combo brings this one alive. The kale will keep you healthy. What a great snack!

Strawberry Blast

1 cup frozen red/dark grapes
1 cup frozen strawberries
1 cup Kale(or raw collard greens)
1 cup apple juice
1cup water

ADD INGREDIENTS TO BLENDER AND BLEND AT HIGH SPEED FOR ONE MINUTE.

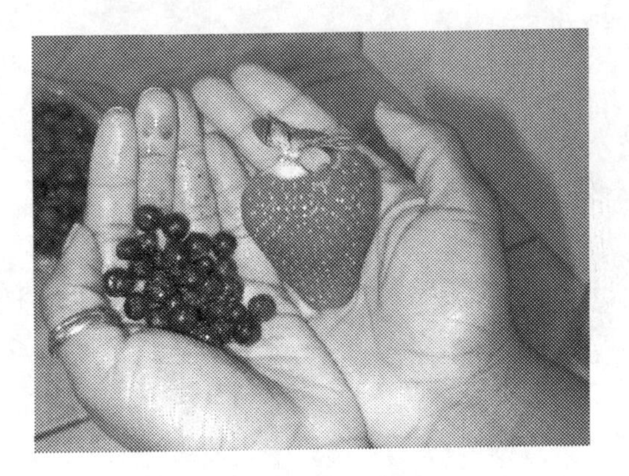

Notes: ______________________________

____

____

____

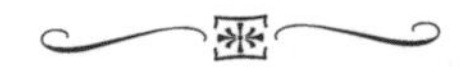

PUNCH IT UP:

Add ¼ tsp of cinnamon for flavor and anti-inflammatory aid!
Add 1tsp-1TBSN of olive oil to create a digestive aid!
Add 1 TBSPN of honey of ENERGY!
Substitute soy milk or skim or nut milk for a variation!

SUPER EFFECTIVE HEALING: Use water instead of apple juice and add one serving of spirulina powder and wheatgrass powder (or wheatgrass shot).

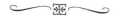

WHAT EXCITES ME ABOUT THIS RECIPE: This one tastes flavorful, the grapes are full of anti-cancerous anti-inflammatory nutrients. The strawberries are anti-cancerous and anti-inflammatory also. That means this delicious drink improves the following conditions: cancer, arthritis, IBS, diabetes, Multiple Sclerosis, Lupus and many other inflammatory diseases. Always consult your physician. This one fights tumors and promotes overall health. So there . . . . remember that as you go on with your day! Dr. William Li advises the use of anti-inflammatory fruit and vegetables to improve angiogenesis explained impressively at this website: http://www.ted.com/talks/william_li.html

Strawberry/Banana

1 cup frozen strawberries
1banana
1 cup kale (or raw collard greens)
12 oz apple juice

ADD INGREDIENTS TO BLENDER AND BLEND AT HIGH SPEED FOR ONE MINUTE.

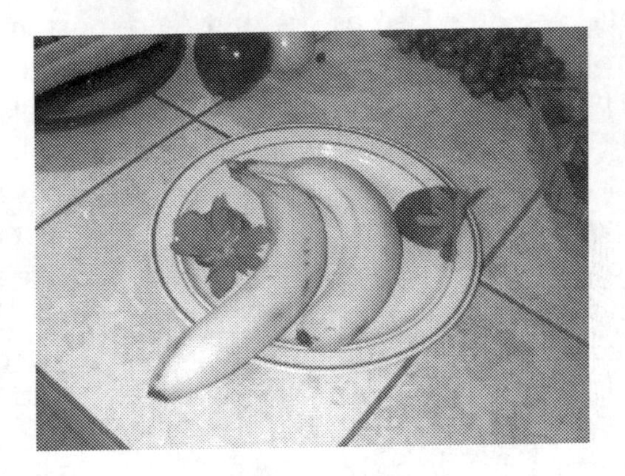

Notes:____

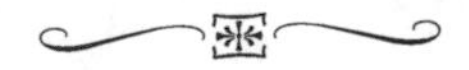

PUNCH IT UP:

Add ¼ tsp of cinnamon for flavor and anti-inflammatory aid!
Add 1tsp-1TBSN of olive oil to create a digestive aid!
Add 1 TBSPN of honey of ENERGY!
Substitute soy milk or skim or nut milk for a variation!

SUPER EFFECTIVE HEALING: Use water instead of apple juice and add one serving of spirulina powder and wheatgrass powder (or wheatgrass shot).

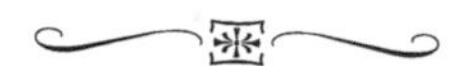

WHAT EXCITES ME ABOUT THIS RECIPE: This tastes like a shake! It is soo good and is totally anti-cancerous and anti-inflammatory. Keep it RAW!!! ADD CINNAMON. Oz EATING HEALTHY IS FUN AND EASY!

Green Strawberries

1 cup frozen strawberries
1 cup kale(or raw collard greens)
4oz apple juice
4 oz of water

ADD INGREDIENTS TO BLENDER AND BLEND AT HIGH SPEED FOR ONE MINUTE.

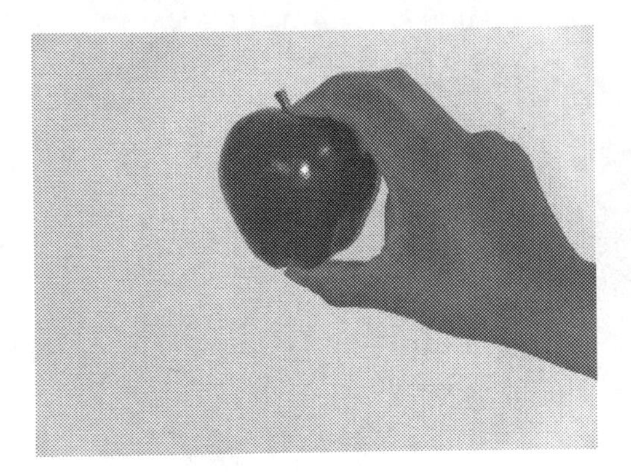

Notes: ____

____

____

____

____

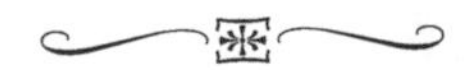

PUNCH IT UP:

Add ¼ tsp of cinnamon for flavor and anti-inflammatory aid!
Add 1tsp-1TBSN of olive oil to create a digestive aid!
Add 1 TBSPN of honey of ENERGY!
Substitute soy milk or skim or nut milk for a variation!

SUPER EFFECTIVE HEALING: Use water instead of apple juice and add one serving of spirulina powder and wheatgrass powder (or wheatgrass shot).

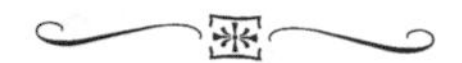

WHAT EXCITES ME ABOUT THIS RECIPE: This is another great tasting shake. The strawberries are rich in anti-oxidants and are cancer fighting fruit. Strawberries help with appetite control and fat-fighting as well. Berries and Kale shake—YUMMY!

Fiber Squared

[illegible]ks of celery (cut into 2 inch pieces)
[illegible]artered Apple
5 oz of apple juice
5 oz water
¼ teaspoon of vanilla

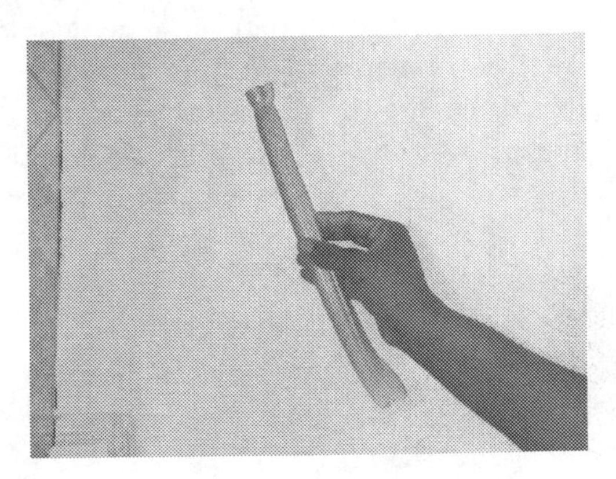

Notes: ______________________________

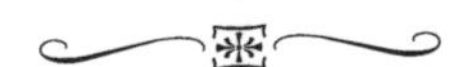

PUNCH IT UP:

Add ¼ tsp vanilla for flavor.
Add ¼ tsp of cinnamon for flavor and anti-inflammatory aid!
Add 1tsp-1TBSN of olive oil to create a digestive aid!
Add 1 TBSPN of honey of ENERGY!
Substitute soy milk or skim or nut milk for a variation!

SUPER EFFECTIVE HEALING: Use water instead of apple juice and add one serving of spirulina powder and wheatgrass powder (or wheatgrass shot).

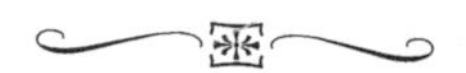

WHAT EXCITES ME ABOUT THIS RECIPE: This recipe is first of all tasty. There is so much fiber in this one that it will help your digestion right away. If you add olive oil it will help rid excess gas effectively also. The celery helps by having an anti-oxidant effect. It is good for cancer conditions. It is good for indigestion, bad breath, cancer fungal infections and gout. Celery also has a pain killing side-effect and aids in headache relief! This dynamic duo is a great breakfast drink or snack through out the day!

Carrot Power

2 carrots (cut into 2 inch segments)
12 oz apple cider
4 oz water
½ tspn vanilla
¼ tspn of cinnamon

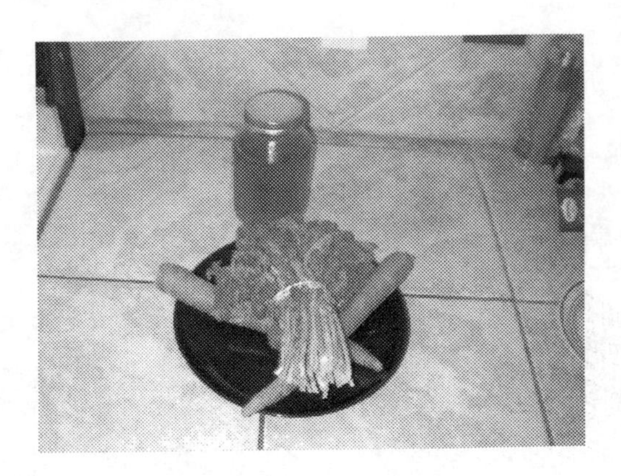

Notes: ____________________

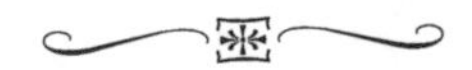

PUNCH IT UP:

Add ¼ tsp of vanilla flavoring for more flavor!
Add 1tsp-1TBSN of olive oil to create a digestive aid!
Substitute soy milk or skim or nut milk for a creamy variation!

SUPER EFFECTIVE HEALING: Use water instead of apple juice and add one serving of spirulina powder and wheatgrass powder (or wheatgrass shot).

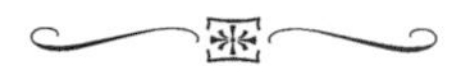

WHAT EXCITES ME ABOUT THIS RECIPE: The carrots are known to help us in so many ways: improves vision, lower cholesterol, strengthens heart, anti-cancerous, improves skin, regulates digestion, improves teeth and gums, prevent stroke, PHEW! Combined with anti-oxidants health building effect of apple juice this is a dynamic snack!

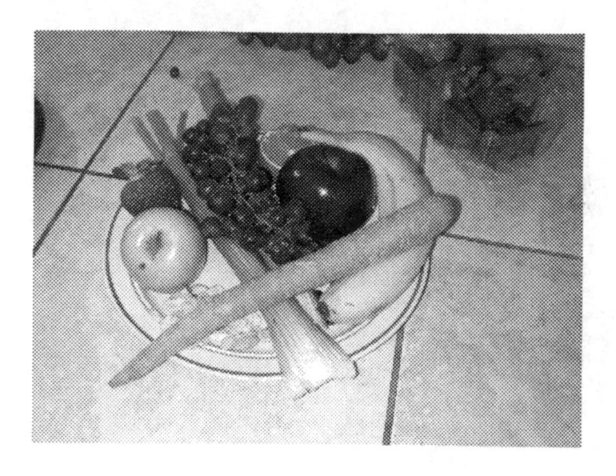

Banana-Orange Kale

1 banana
1 seedless orange/ 2 tangerines
1 cup of kale (or raw collard greens)
12 oz of apple juice

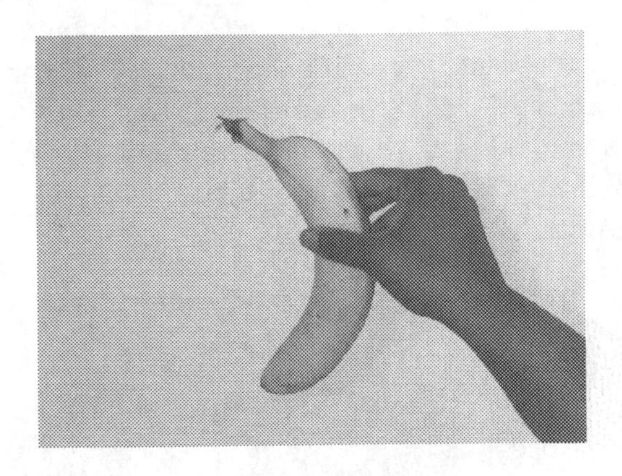

Notes:

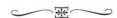

PUNCH IT UP:

Add ¼ tsp of vanilla flavoring for more flavor!
Add 1tsp-1TBSN of olive oil to create a digestive aid!
Add 1 TBSPN of honey of ENERGY!
Substitute soy milk or skim or nut milk for a variation!

SUPER EFFECTIVE HEALING: Use water instead of apple juice and add one serving of spirulina powder and wheatgrass powder (or wheatgrass shot).

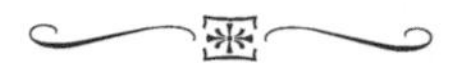

WHAT EXCITES ME ABOUT THIS RECIPE: It has oranges and kale which are classified as having anti-angiogenic effects. That means that these fruit are anti-cancerous; anti-diabetes, anti-tumor building, anti-IBS, anti-Lupus; anti-Multiple Sclerosis, OK in short anti-any inflammatory disease! What a great drink.

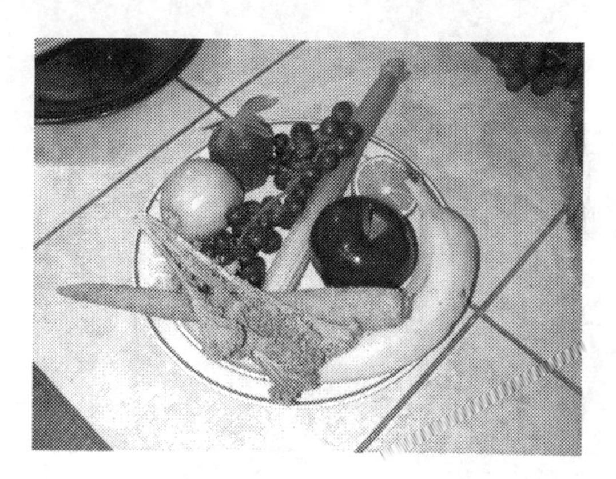

Blue dream

½ cup frozen blueberries
1 banana
5 oz apple juice
5 oz water
¼ tspn cinnamon

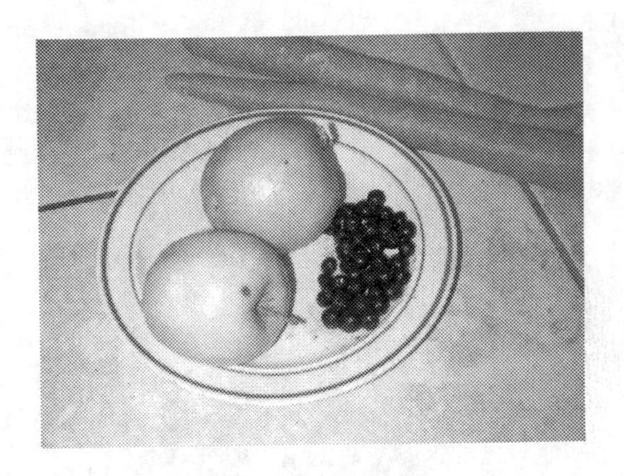

Notes:

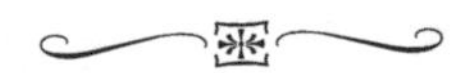

PUNCH IT UP:

Add 1tsp-1TBSN of olive oil to create a digestive aid!
Add 1 TBSPN of honey of ENERGY!
Substitute soy milk or skim or nut milk for a variation!

SUPER EFFECTIVE HEALING: Use water instead of apple juice and add one serving of spirulina powder and wheatgrass powder (or wheatgrass shot).

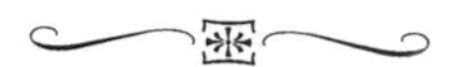

WHAT EXCITES ME ABOUT THIS RECIPE: Blueberries are very antioxidant and anti-angiogenic and they are high in phyto-nutrients that are known to reduce inflammation.

Kale and Berries

½ cup frozen blueberries
½ cup frozen strawberries
1 cup kale (or raw collard greens)
8 oz apple juice
2 oz water

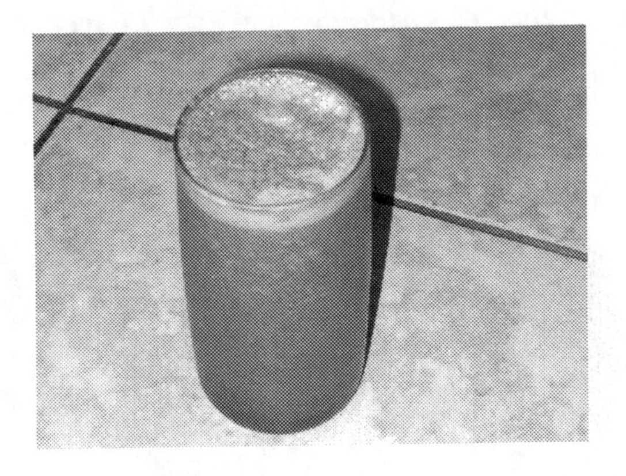

Notes: ______________________________

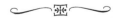

PUNCH IT UP:

Add 1 TBSP of honey for extra energy!
Add ¼ tsp of vanilla flavoring for more flavor!
Add 1tsp-1TBSN of olive oil to create a digestive aid!
Substitute soy milk or skim or nut milk for a creamy variation!

SUPER EFFECTIVE HEALING: Use water instead of apple juice and add one serving of spirulina juice and wheatgrass powder (or wheatgrass shot).

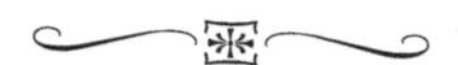

WHAT EXCITES ME ABOUT THIS RECIPE: Everything in this recipe is anti-inflammatory! This one works faster for me than any medicine! This one takes swelling away from my face in the matter of hours. It was from drinking smoothies like these that helped me rediscover my face! My youthful features and glow re-appeared.

Banana/Berry Dream

One Banana
½ cup of frozen strawberries
½ cup of frozen blueberries
1 Tbsp of peanut butter
8oz apple juice
4 oz ice water
¼ tsp cinnamon

Blend for one minute
Serves 3

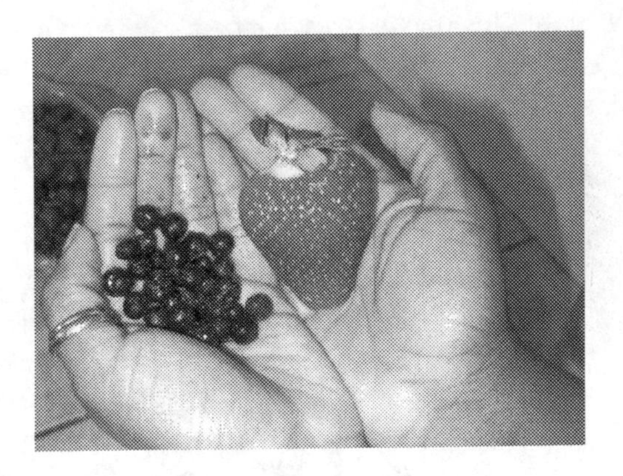

Notes: ______________________________

____

____

____

____

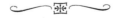

PUNCH IT UP:

Add 1 TBSP of honey for extra energy!
Add ¼ tsp of vanilla flavoring for more flavor!
Add 1tsp-1TBSP of olive oil to create a digestive aid!
Substitute soy milk or skim or nut milk for a creamy variation!

SUPER EFFECTIVE HEALING: Use water instead of apple juice and add one serving of spirulina powder and wheatgrass powder (or wheatgrass shot).

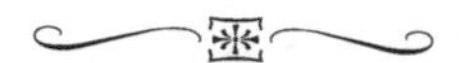

WHAT EXCITES ME ABOUT THIS RECIPE: This tastes like a dream! It is completely anti-inflammatory. This means it helps improve many conditions. This is great for dessert! These all healthy natural ingredients can help you start your day great or end it well also!!

Benefits of Ingredients

I researched the benefits of the produce I add to my drinks. Here's some information for you to use.
By incorporating green leafy vegetables into my diet my health improved in many different ways. Green leafy vegetables such as collard greens, kale, mustard greens and spinach (to name a few) increase my intake of chlorophyll and chlorella by significant amounts. The effects are improved digestion, heavy metal detoxification, increased calcium intake among many benefits.

People that choose to eat "green leafies" regularly have a lower rate of cancer; heart disorders; hypertention; osteoporosis!

You could just take vitamins, you say! By eating green leafies and thoroughly masticating them you receive effective "absorbable nutrients". Try it along with your vitamins.

http://www.eatgreenforlife.com/

Many nutrients that give fruit their color also make these fruit beneficial for us. Blue and purple fruits and veggies have an impressive amount of anthocyanins and phenolics. These are strong antioxidant compounds that help with anti-aging.

Generally, green vegetables decease risk of cancer and are anti-oxidant. Some of these green veggies help flush carcinogens out of your system therefore reducing the risk of many diseases.

As a rule white brown and yellow vegetables lower cholesterol; strengthen hearts; and reduce the likelihood of some cancers.

Yellow and orange fruit and vegetables contain compounds and antioxidants such as vitamin C. These are vital elements that contribute to healthy vision, reliable heart, durable immune system, and decreased cancer risks.

http://healthscienceresearch.com

Here are some benefits of the fruits and vegetables that are in your smoothies. These benefits can be found WWW.livestrong.com Unless otherwise mentioned.

APPLES

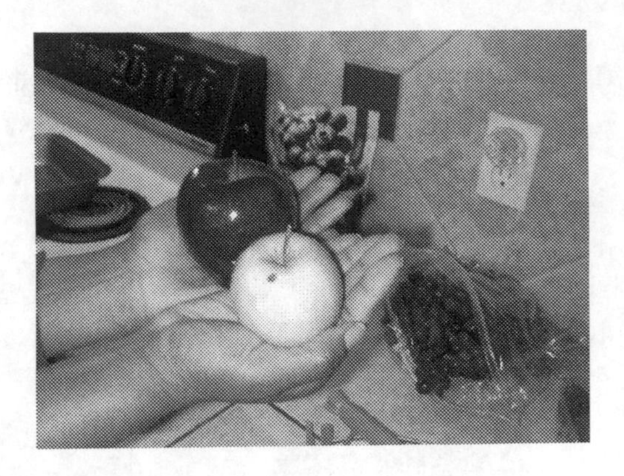

Bone Protection

Phloridzin (found only in apples) protects women from osteoporosis during post-menopausal stages and in known for increasing “bone density. Apples are loaded with Boron that strengthens bones.

Asthma Help

Studies show that children with asthma that drink apple juice daily experienced less wheezing than children who drink apple juice only once per month. Another study showed that children of mothers who eat many apples daily have less asthma than mothers who do not eat apples as often.

Alzheimer’s Prevention

A study on mice that eat mice and have an increased amount of quercetin are less likely to develop Alzheimers Disease.

Lower Cholesterol

Eating at least twice daily can significantly reduce cholesterol levels.

Breast Cancer Prevention
According to Cornell University a study using rats showed that breast cancer could be significantly reduced by simply eating three apples a day!

Colon Cancer Prevention
One study found that rats could reduce the rate of colon cancer by 43% by eating apple skins. Research studies show that the pectin in apples also reduces the risk of colon cancer.

Liver cancer can also be decreased by eating apple skins.

The pectin in apples supplies galacturonic acid to the body which increases diabetics ability to manage blood sugar.

A Brazilian study found that dieting women who ate three apples or pears daily lost more weight.

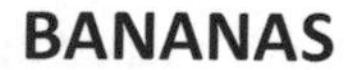

BANANAS

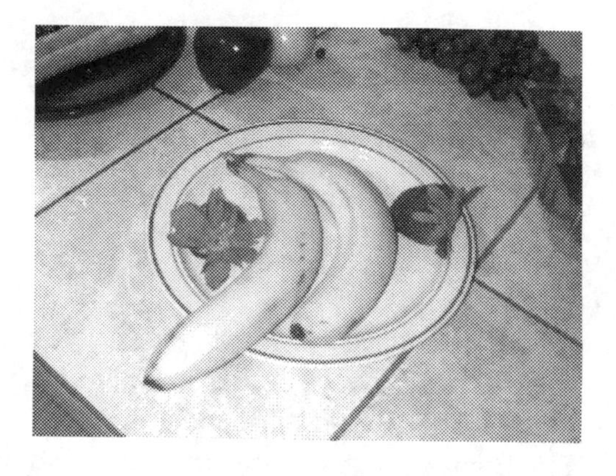

We all eat bananas whether in bread or in cereal. Bananas are exceptional in smoothies and can mask the flavor of bitter greens.

Diet
One banana has approximately 10% of the RDA of dietary fiber and only about 100 calories. Bananas are great for digestion.

Studies show that the high amounts of potassium in bananas (over 13% of the RDA) can lower one's blood pressure, which can decrease chances of atherosclerosis, heart attack and stroke.

Bone Health
In addition to lowering blood pressure, potassium and calcium also strengthen bone density. The typical diet causes calcium to be lost through the urine, which threatens blood clotting, healthy muscle development, and normal nervous system function.

Increased Nutrient Absorption
The potassium in bananas maintain the proper levels of calcium in our body. Bananas also contain high amount of nutrient absorbing compounds that help us absorb calcium. Bananas increase the body's ability to absorb nutrients.

Healthy Digestive Tract
Bananas are often used as a light meal when recovering from stomach ailments and digestive sickness. Bananas are soothing and provide vitamins and minerals while promoting a soothing and easy-to-digest meal.

Stomach Problems
Bananas shield the stomach and intricate digestive system in two ways. Firstly, they produce mucus in the stomach, which shields against stomach acids. Secondly, bananas possess inhibitors, that break down bacteria in the stomach that cause ulcers. (Also, studies show that inhibitors found in bananas also halt the production of certain cells and viruses, including HIV.)

Cancer Prevention

A study by the Internal Journal of Cancer reports that the chance of developing "kidney cancer is decreased by daily consumption of fruits and vegetables—especially bananas. The risk of developing kidney cancer for female subjects decreases by 50% when women eat bananas at least four times a week.

Vitamin B6

One banana has an impressive 34% of recommended vitamin B6, which fills many important funtions in the body's. For example, the B6 in bananas acts as an anti-inflammatory food that helps stave off heart disease and type II diabetes. B6 also contributes to the health of the lymphoid glands. They ensure the production of healthy white blood cells that shield the body from infections. Finally, the vitamin B6 in bananas serves as an integral part in cell development and healthy neurological system functioning.

BLUEBERRIES

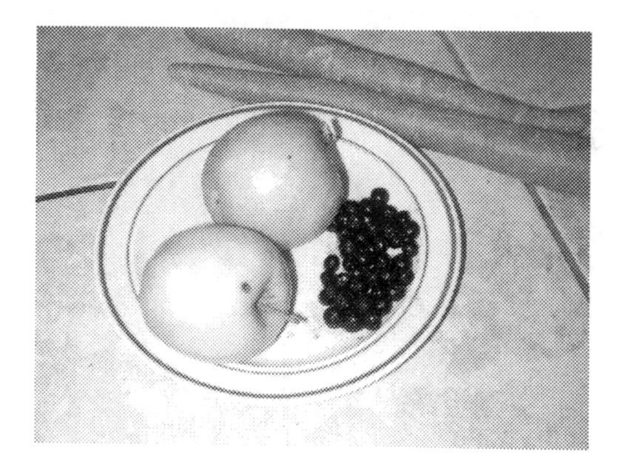

Many nutrients in blueberries are proven to be cancer fighters, such as resveratrol, flavanols, and anthocyanins.

Alzheimer's Disease

Studies show that consumption of blueberries may help decrease or alleviate the cognitive degeneration associated with Alzheimer's disease. Researchers found that the drinking of wild blueberry juice improved memory in the aged.

Hepatitis C

Researchers have discovered that a chemical in blueberry leaves can inhibit the progression of disease in people infected with hepatitis C.

Heart Disease

The antioxidants and many other important nutrients alive in blueberries contribute to a durable heart and overall cardiovascular system.

Urinary Tract Infections

Researchers have found blueberries to be helpful in preventing urinary tract infections by slowing the growth of infection causing bacteria.

Cholesterol

Animal studies have found that a compound in blueberries may lower cholesterol as effectively as prescription drugs without the side effects.

Blood Pressure

According to researchers blood pressure may be lowered and regulated by regular consumption of blueberries and blueberry juice.

Antioxidants

Blueberries have an enormous amount of antioxidants and anti-inflammatory agents that reduce discomfort and alleviate inflammation regarding inflammatory diseases such as Arthritis, Lupus, IBS etc.

CARROTS

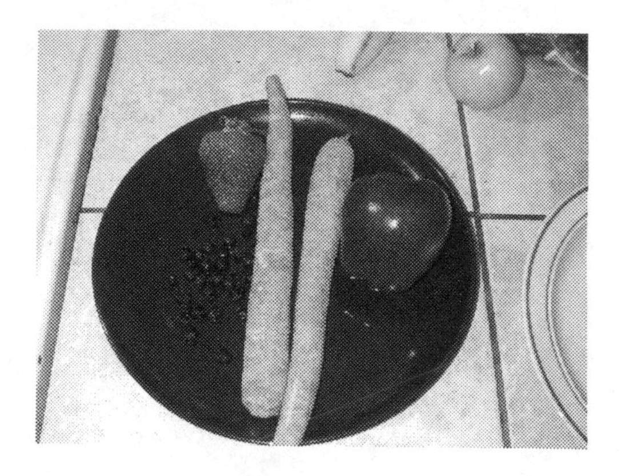

Of course, carrots are great for your eyes; but, here are more benefits of this common vegetable.

1.) Carrots have energizing properties.
2.) They cleanse the system of impurities—improving digestion.
3.) Carrots contain calcium, which benefits the skin, hair, and bones.
4.) This vegetable may help in the treatment of eye problems.
5.) They are useful in the treatment of respiratory conditions.
6.) Often carrots may help relieve skin disorders.
7.) Also, they may help to overcome many glandular disorders.
8.) Carrots may help to regulate the menstrual cycle.
9.) They are great for your anti-inflammatory diet.
10.) They are also antiseptic.

Caution: Eating an excessive amount of carrots may turn your skin orange. Also avoid eating large quantities during pregnancy.

Recommendations: Drink fresh, raw carrot juice daily to energize and cleanse the body.

CELERY

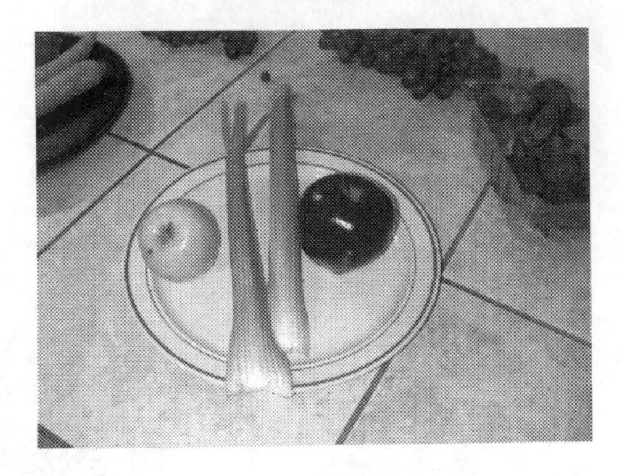

According to www.healthdiaries.com Celery is strengthening for the immune system. The calcium, magnesium, and potassium in celery also helps regulate blood pressure. The pthalides in celery may also lower cholesterol by increasing bile acid secretion. Celery contains coumarins which have been shown to be effective in the prevention of cancer.

Celery has a diuretic effect. Directly related it also has potassium and sodium that help flush the system. That effects also consequently reduces inflammation!

CINNAMON

- I love cinnamon. And for good reason. Here's some useful information on the benefits of cinnamon!! I read Michelle Schoffor's "10 Surprising Health Benefits of Cinnamon" (12-28-2011). Here is what I found interesting. (http://www.care2.com/greenliving/10-surprising-health-benefits-of-cinnamon.html#ixzz2Kbw2Rkhr)

1. Researchers found that cinnamon **balances blood sugar**, making it a viable choice for diabetics and hypoglycemics. It also regulates energy levels and moods.
2. Cinnamon **decreases LDL cholesterol levels**; therefore; reducing the risk of cardiovascular disease.
3. Cinnamon has natural anti-infectious agents. Researchers have found that cinnamon has natural anti-septic effect resulting in decreasing harmful bacteria reactions leading to various infections in the body.
4. Cinnamon **decreases pain linked to arthritis**. Cinnamon has been shown in studies to reduce inflammation caused by arthritis.
5. Research at the University of Texas, published in the journal *Nutrition and Cancer*, shows that cinnamon **may reduce the growth of cancer cells**, holding promise for cancer prevention.
6. It preserves food.
7. Cinnamon has fiber and small amounts of essential minerals.
8. Cinnamon aids with female menstrual aches and pains.
9. **Regular use of Cinnamon increases and balances hormones that lead to infertility.**
10. Research shows that cinnamon has been significantly effective in managing various neurodegenerative diseases, including: **Alzheimer's disease, Parkinson's disease, Multiple Sclerosis, Brain Tumors, and Meningitis**, according to research at the Cytokine Research Laboratory, Department of Experimental Therapeutics, The University of Texas. Their research shows that cinnamon reduces chronic inflammation linked with these neurological disorders.

COLLARD GREENS

Please enjoy the information that I gathered at http:// www.nutrition-and-you.com. Deliciously nutritious collard leaves are low calorie and no fat. The green leaves contain an impressive amount of fiber. There is some insoluble dietary fiber that helps control LDL cholesterol levels and serve as defense against hemorrhoids, constipation and even colon cancer diseases. Fresh collard leaves have an abundant amount of vitamin-C! Vitamin-C is an effective anti-oxidant that offers protection against free radical injury and flu-like viral infections. Ward off a cold!

GRAPES

Grapes are terrific for decreasing inflammation. Grapes improve skin texture and skin condition. Grapes are great for the digestion and relieve constipation. Grapes are chock full of resveratrol-meaning grapes have powerful anti-oxidants! Grapes taste wonderful! Grapes have regenerative power that have been used to fight cancer!

People go on grape fasts to detox their kidney and liver.

"Let food be thy medicine"-Hippocrates!

HONEY

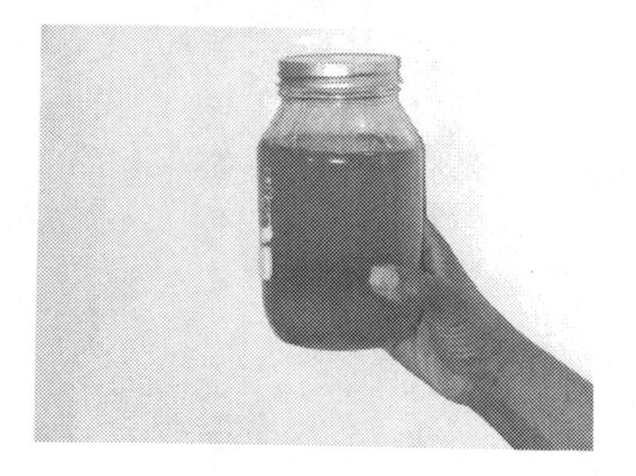

Here are some health benefits of honey: You have to love the flavor!

Cancer Prevention

Honey is energy supplying, antiseptic, anti-inflammatory. Research is undecided of how effective it is for cancer prevention alone. It has had significant effects on cancer prevention in combination with various prescribed treatments.

Antioxidants

Research shows that daily consumption of honey raises anti-oxidants in the blood. It provides antioxidants that are unique of honey.

Immune System Support

Honey stimulates the immune system. Processed honey is not as effective as raw honey. This may be the reason people add it to tea when they are sick!

Boosts Energy

Honey has natural sugars and carbohydrates contributing to that natural "lift" that is experienced from a small dose.

Antiseptic

It is said that honey can be applied topically to wounds for antiseptic effect and quick healing.

Antiviral & Antibacterial

Honey's anti-bacterial, antiseptic nature make it the perfect for flu and cold season. Treating sore throat to runny nose with effectiveness.

Antifungal

Honey applied topically can treat skin diseases such as ringworm effectively when applied topically.

Healthiest Sweetener

In studies with patients with Type 2 diabetes that honey is a safer choice than refined cane sugar. Some have even used this substance in small doses without affecting their sugar negatively at all.

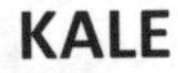

KALE

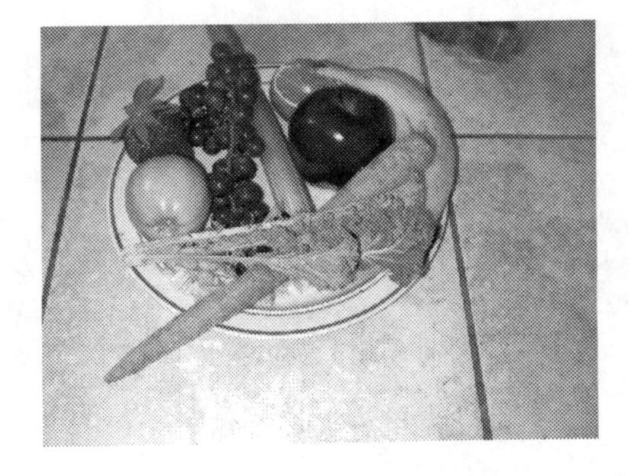

I love kale. I eat it in soups; on sandwiches; in smoothies etc. Here's some benefits I gathered and some I found on www.

healthdiaries.com. Kale is tasty and is anti-inflammatory. It helps me so with my digestion. Read and discover the benefits.

Diet and Digestion

One cup of kale has very low calories (less than 40 calories a cup) and no fat, which makes it a great snacking food. Surprisingly, 8 oz contains nearly 1/5 of the RDA of dietary fiber, which ensures healthy digestion, alleviates constipation, reduces blood sugar and quells overeating. Finally, has glucosinolate isothiocyanate (ITC) that combats detrimental bacterial growth that causes stomach conditions and gastric cancer.

Antioxidants

Carotenoids and flavonoids make kale outshine many other greens. This dynamic duo inadvertently protects us from stress! Key flavonoids flavonoids in kale prove to combat against the development of cancer. Kale has many anti-oxidants that battle against carcinogens and oxidation of cells. Oxidation leads to premature aging and disease.

Anti-Inflammatory

The body's inflammatory process is regulated by omega 3 oils—another plus for kale, chalking up with over 10% omega 3 oil. Kale is full of vitamin K: spearheading it to be a leader in managing inflammation! That means it is good at controlling inflammatory disease symptoms: Multiple Sclerosis Symptoms, Lupus Symptoms, Arthritis Symptoms, IBS symptoms, etc.

Cancer

Kale manages inflammation terrifically! Most of us have cancer cells in our body. They only become a problem once they inflame and become active according to Dr. Willam Li.

By eating kale inflammation is reduced and cancer may be prevented.

Cardiovascular Support
Kale has high fiber that chemically reacts in our system and lowers the detrimental effects of cholesterol.

ORANGES

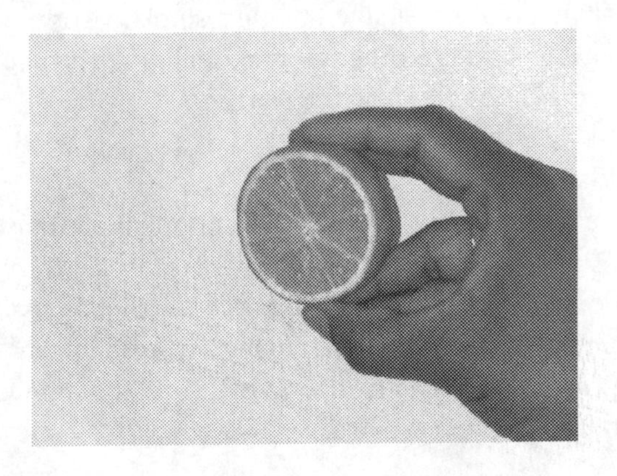

Oranges are great. They are chock full of anti-oxidants. They are anti-inflammatory, mineral-laden, anti-cancerous, nutritious treats! They contain vitamin C, A, potassium, magnesium, calcium. They shield against heart disease; relieve constipation; purify blood; protect against viral infections; protect against kidney diseases; strengthen bones and teeth. Another great fruit that repairs and prevents!

PEANUTBUTTER

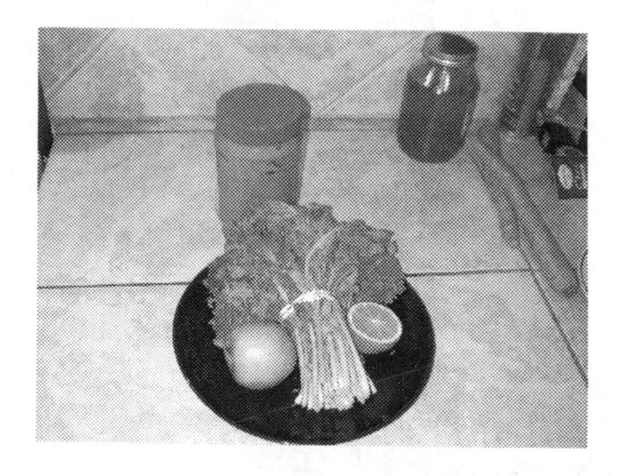

Be careful when choosing your peanutbutter or nut butter. Often there are hidden sugars and salts. Read the label. You want no added sugars and no added salts; no high fructose corn syrup. You can add your own sea salt and honey to your satisfaction. Peanut butter has plenty fiber and protein. It has a great amount of omega three oils—similar to olive oil. I use it in my smoothies with fruit and veggies as a complete protein. It is great to treat constipation. The oils are great for the skin also.

STRAWBERRIES

Strawberries are extremely anti-inflammatory. They are loaded with vitamin C. Which helps with immunity and eye strength. They contain manganese which helps with immunity, degeneration recovery, and healthy bones. They fight cancer. Again they help with any inflammatory disease. The anti-oxidant anti-angiogenic anti-inflammatory nature of this fruit makes it perfect for skin and hair.

SPIRULINA

Spirulina is a sea mineral providing proteins and nutrients that are not easily found in such quantities in other vegetables. Spirulina boasts of having impressive amounts of chlorophyll and chlorella that has been proven to alleviate many chronic disease symptoms.(www.NOW.com)

WHEATGRASS

Wheatgrass has chlorophyll. This ingredient has proven to be effective helping people recovery from various chronic diseases. Dr. Ann Whigmore and her therapy teams have been helping people triumph successfully over chronic diseases utilizing wheatgrass! (www.wheatgrass kits.com)

The skinny on SUGAR

I have included the following truncated list as a reminder of how important it is to remove sugar from your diet if you are expecting to heal! Dr. Appleton has included quite a bit of supportive information in her book. Using processed diet drinks can be extremely detrimental to your health as well. If you expect to heal you must remove processed sugar from your diet for optimal results. (146 Reasons Why Sugar Is Ruining Your Health by Nancy Appleton, Ph.D.)

I included the top 35 reasons here. Dr. Nancy Appleton has researched and she states that many diseases CAN be caused by sugar. I will list the diseases and health risks that sugar could cause. (There other environmental/genetic factors that also may affect the development of these conditions and diseases as well.)

1. Immune system suppression
2. Mineral imbalance in the body
3. Hyperactivity, anxiety, difficulty concentrating, and crankiness in children
4. Triglyceride imbalance
5. Bacterial infection and/or infectious diseases
6. Tissue elasticity loss
7. High density lipoproteins reduction
8. Probable chromium deficiency
9. Ovarian cancer
10. Fasting Glucose increase
11. Copper deficiency
12. Calcium and magnesium absorption interference
13. Eyesight weakness.
14. Neurotransmitter imbalance
15. Hypoglycemia.
16. Acidic digestive tract
17. Adrenaline level imbalance in children
18. Functional bowel disease due to sugar malabsorbtion
19. Premature aging
20. Alcoholism
21. Tooth decay
22. Obesity
23. Risk of Crohn's disease, and ulcerative colitis
24. Gastric or duodenal ulcers conditions
25. Arthritis
26. Asthma
27. Yeast infections
28. Gallstones.
29. Heart disease
30. Appendicitis
31. Multiple Sclerosis
32. Hemorrhoids
33. Varicose veins
34. Birth control pill complications
35. Periodontal disease

A Word about Exercise

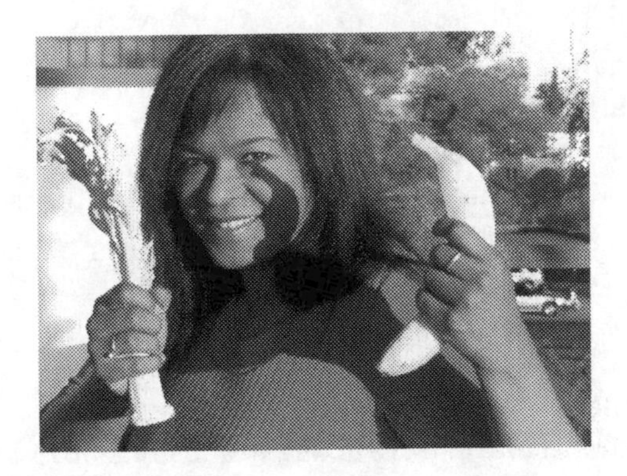

I knew by exercising, I would stimulate or increase my Human Growth Hormone; thus preparing my body to heal rapidly as a child would. (msrecoverydiet.com). That is why I quickly incorporated walking into my exercise regime.

A Cambridge University study showed that jogging 2-3 times a week stimulates new brain interaction. That new interaction effect memory retention and analytical and problem-solving skills as well. These new brain cell interactions improve overall health and slow down the degenerative effect of old age.

Researchers have found that a compound called "noggin" is released while vigorously exercising. This helps out brain to develop. It was believed that no further significant brain development happened after old age; but, researchers have found new information. Good for us!

Notes:

Notes:

Notes:

Notes:

Notes: